Aa-32 Energizer

Erik Kerfoot

ALKALINE

How do basic eating regimens function? Research shows that diets comprising of profoundly soluble food varieties — new vegetables, products of the soil plant-based wellsprings of protein, for instance — bring about a more basic pee pH level, which safeguards sound cells and equilibrium fundamental mineral levels. This can be particularly significant for ladies doing discontinuous fasting and additionally following the keto diet, as chemical levels can be modified.

Basic weight control plans (otherwise called the antacid debris counts calories) have been displayed to help:

forestall plaque development in veins

prevent calcium from collecting in pee

forestall kidney stones

construct more grounded bones

diminish muscle squandering or fits

furthermore, considerably more

What Is A Soluble Eating routine?

A soluble eating regimen is one that is planned to assist with adjusting the blood pH level of the liquids in your body, including your blood and pee.

This diet goes by a few unique names, including:

the basic debris diet

basic corrosive eating routine

corrosive debris diet

pH diet

Dr. Sebi's basic eating routine (Dr. Sebi was a botanist who made a plant-based diet form)

Your pH is to not set in stone by the mineral thickness of the food varieties you eat. Every single living creature and living things on Earth rely upon keeping up with proper pH levels, and it's not unexpected said that illness and turmoil can't flourish in a body that has a reasonable pH.

The standards of the corrosive debris speculation assist with making up the fundamentals of the antacid eating routine. As per research distributed in Diary of Bone and Mineral Exploration, "The corrosive debris speculation sets that protein and grain food varieties, with a low potassium consumption, produce an eating routine corrosive burden, net corrosive discharge (NAE), expanded pee calcium, and arrival of calcium from the skeleton, prompting osteoporosis."

The basic eating routine expects to keep this from occurring via cautiously thinking about food pH levels trying to restrict dietary corrosive admission.

Albeit a few specialists could not thoroughly concur with this assertion, virtually all concur that human existence requires a firmly controlled pH level of the blood of around

7.365-7.4. As Forbe's Magazine puts it, "Our bodies take uncommon measures to keep up with safe pH levels."

Your pH can go between 7.35 to 7.45 relying upon the hour of day, your eating routine, what you last ate and when you last went to the washroom. Assuming you foster electrolyte awkward nature and as often as possible eat such a large number of acidic food varieties — otherwise known as corrosive debris food varieties — your body's changing pH level can result in expanded "acidosis."

Indeed what Does "pH Level" Mean?

What we call pH is short for the capability of hydrogen. It's a proportion of the corrosiveness or alkalinity of the body's liquids and tissues.

It's deliberate on a scale from 0 to 14. The more acidic an answer is, the lower its pH. The more basic, the higher the number is.

A pH of around 7 is viewed as impartial, yet since the ideal human body will in general be around 7.4, we believe the best pH to be one that is marginally basic.

These levels additionally fluctuate all through the body, with the stomach the most acidic area. Indeed, even extremely little modifications in the pH level of different life forms can create significant issues.

For instance, because of ecological worries, for example, expanding CO2 testimony, the pH of the sea has dropped from 8.2 to 8.1, and different daily routine structures experiencing in the sea have extraordinarily endured.

The pH level is likewise vital for developing plants, and in this manner it extraordinarily influences the mineral substance of the food sources we eat. Minerals in the sea, soil and human body are utilized as cradles to keep up with ideal pH levels, so when sharpness rises, minerals fall.

How a Basic Eating routine Functions

Here is some foundation on corrosive/alkalinity in the human eating routine, in addition to central issues about how basic weight control plans can be gainful:

Scientists accept that with regards to the complete corrosive heap of the human eating regimen, "there have been extensive changes from agrarian civic establishments to the present." Following the horticultural insurgency and afterward mass industrialization of our food supply throughout the course of recent years, the food we eat has essentially less potassium, magnesium and chloride, alongside more sodium, contrasted with diets of the past.

Ordinarily, the kidneys keep up with our electrolyte levels (those of calcium, magnesium, potassium and sodium). At the point when we're presented to excessively acidic substances, these electrolytes are utilized to battle acridity.

As per the Diary of Natural Wellbeing audit referenced before, the proportion of potassium to sodium in a great many people's eating regimens has changed emphatically. Potassium used to dwarf sodium by 10:1, yet at this point the proportion has dropped to 1:3. Individuals eating a "Standard American Eating regimen" presently consume three fold the amount of sodium as potassium overall! This contributes extraordinarily to a soluble climate in our bodies.

Numerous kids and grown-ups today consume a high-sodium diet that is extremely low in magnesium and potassium, yet in addition cell reinforcements, fiber and fundamental nutrients. Additionally, the average Western eating routine is high in refined fats, basic sugars, sodium and chloride.

These progressions to the human eating regimen have come about in expanded "metabolic acidosis." all in all, the pH levels of many individuals' bodies are as of now not ideal. On top of this, many are experiencing low supplement admission and issues like potassium and lack of magnesium.

Medical advantages

For what reason is a basic eating routine great for you? Basic food varieties supply significant supplements that assist with halting sped up indications of maturing and a steady loss of organ and cell capabilities.

As made sense of more underneath, basic eating routine advantages might incorporate dialing back degeneration of tissues and bone mass, which can be compromised when an excessive amount of acridity denies us of key minerals.

1. Safeguards Bone Thickness and Bulk

Your admission of minerals assumes a significant part in the turn of events and support of bone designs. Research proposes that the additional alkalizing products of the soil somebody eats, the better security that individual could have from encountering diminished bone strength and muscle squandering as she ages, known as sarcopenia.

A soluble eating regimen can uphold bone wellbeing by adjusting the proportion of minerals that are significant for building bones and keeping up with slender bulk, including calcium, magnesium and phosphate.

The eating routine may likewise assist with further developing creation of development chemicals and vitamin D assimilation, which further safeguards bones as well as alleviating numerous other ongoing infections.

2. Brings down Chance for Hypertension and Stroke

One of the counter maturing impacts of a soluble eating routine is that it diminishes aggravation and causes an expansion in development chemical creation.

This has been displayed to work on cardiovascular wellbeing and deal insurance against normal issues like elevated cholesterol, hypertension (hypertension), kidney stones, stroke and even cognitive decline.

3. Brings down Constant Torment and Irritation

Studies have tracked down an association between a basic eating regimen and diminished degrees of persistent torment. Persistent acidosis has been found to add to constant back torment, migraines, muscle fits, feminine side effects, aggravation and joint agony.

One review led by the General public for Minerals and Minor Components in Germany found that when patients with constant back torment were given a soluble enhancement day to day for a considerable length of time, 76 of 82 patients detailed huge declines in torment as estimated by the "Arhus low back torment rating scale."

4. Supports Nutrient Retention and Forestalls Magnesium Insufficiency

An expansion in magnesium is expected for the capability of many catalyst frameworks and real cycles. Many individuals are lacking in magnesium and subsequently experience heart complexities, muscle torments, cerebral pains, rest inconveniences and tension.

Accessible magnesium is additionally expected to enact vitamin D and forestall lack of vitamin D, which is significant for generally speaking safe and endocrine working.

5. Works on Invulnerable Capability and Potentially Disease Insurance

At the point when cells need an adequate number of minerals to appropriately discard squander or oxygenate the body completely, the entire body endures. Nutrient retention is undermined by mineral misfortune, while poisons and microbes gather in the body and debilitate the safe framework.

Might a soluble eating regimen at any point assist with forestalling disease? While the point is disputable despite everything problematic, research distributed in the English Diary of Radiology tracked down proof that destructive cell demise (apoptosis) was bound to happen in a basic body.

Malignant growth avoidance is accepted to be related with a soluble change in pH because of a modification in electric charges and the arrival of essential parts of proteins. Alkalinity can assist with diminishing irritation and the gamble for sicknesses like malignant growth — in addition to a soluble eating routine has been demonstrated to be more useful for a few chemotherapeutic specialists that require a higher pH to properly work.

6. Can Assist You With keeping a Sound Weight

Albeit the eating routine isn't exclusively centered around fat misfortune, following a soluble eating routine dinner plan for weight reduction can unquestionably help safeguard against stoutness.

Restricting utilization of corrosive framing food varieties and eating more soluble shaping food sources might make it simpler to get thinner because of the eating regimen's capacity to diminish leptin levels and irritation. This influences both your craving and fat consuming skills.

Since basic shaping food sources are calming food sources, devouring a soluble eating regimen allows your body an opportunity to accomplish ordinary leptin levels and feel fulfilled from eating how much calories you truly need.

On the off chance that weight reduction is one of your principal objectives, one of the most mind-blowing ways to deal with attempt is a keto soluble eating routine, which is low in carbs and high in sound fats.

Instructions to Follow

How would you keep your body soluble? Here are a few vital ways to follow a soluble eating regimen:

1. Purchase Natural Soluble Food varieties

Specialists feel that one significant thought concerning eating a soluble eating regimen is to become proficient about what sort of soil your produce was filled in — since leafy foods that are filled in natural, mineral-thick soil will generally be really alkalizing. Research shows that the sort of soil that plants are filled in can altogether impact their nutrient and mineral substance, and that implies not every "soluble food" are made similarly.

The ideal pH of soil for the best by and large accessibility of fundamental supplements in plants is somewhere in the range of 6 and 7. Acidic soils under a pH of 6 might have diminished calcium and magnesium, and soil over a pH of 7 might bring about synthetically inaccessible iron, manganese, copper and zinc.

Soil that is very much turned, naturally maintained and presented to untamed life/eating dairy cattle will in general be the best.

2. Eat More Soluble Food sources and Significantly Less Acidic Food sources

See the rundown beneath of the best basic eating routine food sources, in addition to those to keep away from.

3. Hydrate

Soluble water has a pH of 9 to 11. Refined water is okay to drink. Water sifted with a converse assimilation channel is somewhat acidic, yet it's as yet a far superior choice than faucet water or cleansed filtered water.

Adding pH drops, lemon or lime, or baking soft drink to your water can likewise helps its alkalinity. You can likewise make your own electrolyte drink.

4. (Discretionary) Test Your pH Level

On the off chance that you're interested to realize your pH level prior to executing the tips beneath, you can test your pH by buying strips at your nearby wellbeing food store or drug store. You can quantify your pH with spit or pee.

Your second pee of the morning will give you the best outcomes. You look at the varieties on your test strip to a diagram that accompanies your test strip unit.

During the day, the best opportunity to test your pH is one hour before a dinner and two hours after a feast. Assuming you test with your spit, you need to attempt to remain somewhere in the range of 6.8 and 7.2.

Best Soluble Food varieties

In spite of the fact that you don't need to be severe vegan to eat a high-soluble eating regimen, the eating regimen is for the most part plant-based. Here is a rundown of food varieties to stress most:

New leafy foods advance alkalinity the most. Which are the most ideal decisions; for instance, are bananas soluble? And broccoli? A portion of the top picks incorporate mushrooms, citrus, dates, raisins, spinach, grapefruit, tomatoes, avocado, summer dark radish, hay grass, grain grass, cucumber, kale, jicama, wheatgrass, broccoli, oregano, garlic, ginger, green beans, endive, cabbage, celery, red beet, watermelon, figs and ready bananas.

Every crude food: Preferably attempt to devour a decent part of your produce crude. Uncooked products of the soil are supposed to be biogenic or "nurturing." Cooking food sources drains alkalizing minerals. Increment your admission of crude food sources, and have a go at squeezing or gently steaming products of the soil.

Plant proteins: Almonds, naval force beans, lima beans and most different beans are great decisions.

Soluble water.

Green beverages: Beverages produced using green vegetables and grasses in powder structure are stacked with soluble framing food sources and chlorophyll. Chlorophyll is fundamentally like our own blood and alkalizes the blood.

Different food varieties to eat on a basic eating regimen incorporate fledglings, wheatgrass, kamut, matured soy, as natto or tempeh, and seeds.

Acidic Food sources

What food sources would it be a good idea for you to stay away from while following a basic eating routine eating plan? Acidic food varieties like the accompanying:

High-sodium food varieties: Handled food varieties contain lots of sodium chloride — table salt — which chokes veins and makes sharpness.

Cold cuts and ordinary meats

Handled cereals, (for example, corn chips)

Eggs

Stimulated beverages and liquor

Oats and entire wheat items: All grains, entire or not, make acridity in the body. Americans ingest the greater part of their plant food standard as handled corn or wheat.

Milk: Calcium-rich dairy items cause probably the most elevated paces of osteoporosis. That is on the grounds that they make acridity in the body! At the point when your circulatory system turns out to be excessively acidic, it takes calcium (a more soluble substance) from the unresolved issues to adjust the pH level. The most effective way to forestall osteoporosis is to eat loads of soluble green verdant veggies!

Peanuts and pecans

Pasta, rice, bread and bundled grain items

What different sorts of propensities can cause acridity in your body? The greatest guilty parties include:

Liquor and medication use

High caffeine admission

Anti-toxin abuse

Counterfeit sugars

Ongoing pressure

Declining supplement levels in food varieties because of modern cultivating

Low degrees of fiber in the eating regimen

Absence of activity

Abundance creature meats in the eating routine (from non-grass-took care of sources)

Overabundance chemicals from food varieties, wellbeing and excellence items, and plastics

Openness to synthetic substances and radiation from family chemicals, building materials, PCs, PDAs and microwaves

Food shading and additives

Overexercise

Pesticides and herbicides

Contamination

Unfortunate biting and dietary patterns

Handled and refined food varieties

Shallow relaxing

Versus Paleo Diet

The Paleo diet and basic eating routine share numerous things practically speaking and a ton of similar advantages, for example, brought down risk for supplement lacks, diminished irritation levels, better processing, weight reduction or the board, etc.

A few things that the two share for all intents and purpose incorporate taking out added sugars, lessening admission of favorable to fiery omega-6 unsaturated fats, killing grains and handled carbs, diminishing or dispensing with dairy/milk consumption, and expanding admission of products of the soil.

Nonetheless, there are a few significant interesting points on the off chance that you intend to follow the Paleo diet.

The Paleo diet dispenses with all dairy items, including yogurt and kefir, which can be significant wellsprings of probiotics and minerals for some individuals — in addition to the Paleo diet doesn't necessarily in all cases underline eating natural food varieties or grass-took care of/free roaming meat (and with some restraint/restricted amounts).

Moreover, the Paleo diet will in general incorporate bunches of meat, pork and shellfish, which have their own disadvantages.

Eating such a large number of creature wellsprings of protein overall can really add to sharpness, not alkalinity. Hamburger, chicken, cold cuts, shellfish and pork can add to sulfuric corrosive development in the blood as amino acids are separated. Attempt to get the best quality creature items you can, and differ your admission of protein food varieties to adjust your pH level best.

Recipes

What could a basic eating regimen menu resemble? Utilizing the shopping list above, here are some straightforward and flavorful basic eating regimen recipes to attempt:

Alkalizing Juice Recipe: This green juice utilizes high-soluble food varieties like cucumber, kale and spinach.

50 Astounding Avocado Recipes: All that from mousse to smoothies!

34 Green Smoothie Recipes

Dark Bean Burgers Recipe

Almond Flour Hotcakes or Almond Spread Treats Recipe

Hazard and Incidental effects

Certain food varieties on the "exceptionally acidic rundown" could shock you, like eggs and pecans. These may be acidic in your body, yet don't let that drive you off from eating them. They contain a large group of other medical advantages, similar to cell reinforcements and omega-3 unsaturated fats, which actually makes them important.

We're going for basically a good arrangement. Taking everything into account, it's feasible to turn out to be excessively soluble, and it is both expected and beneficial to have a few acidic food sources.

Our concern is more a question of not taking in enough soluble advancing food varieties as opposed to taking in such a large number of acids from solid, entire food sources. Eat various genuine, entire food sources (particularly vegetables and products of the soil) utilization of bundled things, and you'll be coming.

Last Considerations

What is a basic eating regimen? It's a for the most part plant-based diet that incorporates entire food sources that emphatically affect pH levels of the blood and pee.

Medical advantages of a soluble eating routine can incorporate better heart wellbeing, more grounded bones, diminished torment, help getting in shape and inversion of supplement lacks.

A basic eating plan incorporates a lot of entire products of the soil, crude food sources, green squeezes, beans, and nuts.

Food sources that are acidic and in this manner restricted on a basic eating regimen incorporate high-sodium food varieties, handled grains, an excessive amount of meat and creature protein, added sugars, and customary milk.

With all the gab out there about the basic eating regimen, it's not difficult to feel that perhaps there's something to it. It has a science-y name that rings of science based truth. There are not difficult to-follow records all around the web letting you know what to eat and what to stay away from. Star competitors are building up it. Superstar forces to be reckoned with are on top of it. Perhaps this is the genuine article, correct?

But, as such countless things throughout everyday life, the cases made by devotees of the antacid eating routine aren't really obvious. Furthermore, its guarantee to "hack" your body's capabilities simply doesn't face logical thoroughness.

"With everything taken into account, the basic eating routine can be protected and useful whenever done well," says enrolled dietitian Anthony DiMarino, RD. "This diet can assist with keeping you solid, yet not for the reasons you could think."

DiMarino separates the advantages and disadvantages of this moving eating routine so you can choose if going antacid is ideal for you.

What is the antacid eating routine?

On the off chance that you recollect much from science class, or on the other hand on the off chance that you invest energy keeping a pool or nursery, you may be know all about pH — an estimation of how acidic or essential (basic) an answer is. It's scored on a size of 0 to 14.

A pH of 0 to 6 is acidic.

A pH of 7 is unbiased.

A pH of 8 or higher is essential, or soluble.

The soluble eating regimen depends on the doubtful thought that there are medical advantages to be acquired by moving your body science to the basic side of the scale. Advocates of the eating regimen express that by eating food varieties that are basic, rather than acidic or unbiased, you'll:

Avoid persistent circumstances like osteoporosis and malignant growth.

Increment your energy.

Get thinner.

However, consider this: A few pieces of your body are normally acidic. A few pieces of your body are normally soluble. What's more, there's not actually anything you can do to change that — nor would you truly need to.

"Your body is a shrewd machine. It controls pH very well all alone," DiMarino says. "Our stomachs are extremely acidic, so they can separate food. Our skin has a somewhat acidic pH to safeguard against microscopic organisms. Our lungs and kidneys work to eliminate metabolic waste and keep our body pH where it should be."

Your blood stays at a basic level between around 7.2 and 7.4. Assuming the pH drops out of that reach, it very well may be lethal. Fortunate for us, however, nothing you eat will change your blood pH.

Would it be a good idea for me to attempt the soluble eating routine?

The basic eating regimen underlines picking normal food sources that are by and large really great for you, so somehow or another, it tends to be an advantage to your wellbeing. In any case, it's not without certain destructions.

DiMarino thinks about the advantages and disadvantages.

Expert: Soluble food sources are by and large sound decisions

Not at all like some other trend counts calories (here's taking a gander at you, fruitarians), the soluble eating routine is stuffed brimming with food sources that have high dietary benefit. It confines added sugars and supports keeping away from bundled food sources for new food varieties that are notable for their wellbeing esteem.

"The basic eating routine supports low-handled, entire food sources, which have been displayed to forestall illness in the long haul, so in that regard, it tends to be viewed as a good dieting design," DiMarino notes.

A portion of the mainstays of a basic eating regimen are food varieties we know to be strong staples of a solid eating routine:

Leafy foods organic product juice.

Grains like wild rice, oats and quinoa.

Vegetables.

Non-bland vegetables, as salad greens, broccoli, cabbage and carrots.

Nuts.

Seeds.

These are a portion of the very food sources that examination has demonstrated to be heart-solid, weight reduction well disposed and generally around really great for you. So it makes sense that, indeed, when you make solid, entire food sources the premise of your eating regimen, you can receive some serious wellbeing rewards.

Con: You might pass up protein and different supplements

Protein is vital to help develop and fix muscle, supply supplements to your body and substantially more. In any case, on the off chance that you're sticking near the basic eating routine, numerous normal wellsprings of protein are untouchable.

The soluble eating routine is a plant-based diet. Like a veggie lover diet, it considers no creature proteins, including meats, eggs or dairy. Individuals who follow a vegetarian diet can get adequate supplements from plant-based proteins like:

Lentils.

Soybeans and soy milk.

Tempeh.

Tofu.

The strictest supporters of the soluble eating routine, be that as it may, will say these food sources are acidic or corrosive shaping and ought to be kept away from. Other antacid eating routine adherents take into account limited quantities of plant proteins, from soy or lentils for instance.

"Following an inflexible soluble eating regimen will make it hard to get an adequate number of supplements like protein, iron and calcium," DiMarino alerts. "Low protein can cause loss of bulk. Low iron can cause pallor. What's more, low calcium can be a gamble to your bone wellbeing."

The U.S. Division of Agribusiness suggests:

Grown-up ladies and individuals alloted female upon entering the world (AFAB) consume 5 to 6.5 ounces of protein every day.

Grown-up men and individuals alloted male upon entering the world (AMAB) consume 5.5. to 7 ounces of protein every day.

Con: The basic eating routine can be serious and exorbitant

In the event that you're focused on food obtaining and feast prep (or on the other hand assuming you have an individual cook à la Hollywood sovereignty), a basic eating routine can squeeze into your way of life. In any case, the boundary to passage might be excessively high for certain individuals.

Keeping the appropriate organic products, veggies and grains close by (and new) requires some cautious anticipating your part. Entire, nutritious food varieties aren't promptly accessible to all individuals in all seasons, and their expense can be a boundary. There's even basic water available, sold along with some built-in costs.

"A basic eating routine is innately difficult to follow," DiMarino says. "It centers solely around entire, natural food sources, which can rely upon the season and might be difficult to come by once in a while. These food sources will quite often be more costly and work concentrated. A basic eating regimen can be supportable, yet you should have the option to design it cautiously and guarantee you're meeting your dietary necessities."

While you're following a soluble eating regimen, eating in eateries, getting take-out or snatching a helpful light meal could demonstrate troublesome. Also, not every person has time or involvement with pre-arranging and setting up every dinner and nibble to guarantee ideal nourishment.

Seeing the outcomes

Individuals following the basic eating regimen consistently use what they call a dipstick to break down the pH in their pee to check whether the eating routine is "working." While the facts really confirm that the pH of your pee will change from acidic to soluble on the off chance that you follow an antacid eating routine (and before long, as well), DiMarino says the pH of your pee reflects nothing about the present status of your wellbeing.

"Our pee is an incredible method for disposing of the metabolic waste from what we eat," he says. "Your pee pH reflects what you needed to eat as of late, however it connotes nothing about the nature of your eating regimen or current wholesome status."

Would it be a good idea for me to talk with a specialist about the basic eating routine?

In the event that you're thinking about following the basic eating routine, talk with a specialist or an enlisted dietitian to check whether you would benefit, and examine ways of guaranteeing you're getting every one of the supplements your body needs.

"I would prescribe to anybody attempting to begin another eating regimen, particularly a popular one, to examine it with their medical services supplier," DiMarino says. "They'll have the option to furnish you with an intensive evaluation and proof based techniques to meet your objectives."

Regardless of what you eat, you won't change your body's pH — and that really intends that toward the day's end, the essential commitment of the antacid eating routine did not depend on logical truth.

In the event that you're ready to invest the effort and guarantee you meet your healthful requirements, the antacid eating regimen may actually assist you with getting thinner and avert a few normal ongoing circumstances. Yet, proven techniques like customary activity and a solid, adjusted diet stay the highest quality level — no dipstick-pee-test required.

The pH of water is a significant determinant of its destructiveness, which is essentially a proportion of how horrendous water is toward the metals of water circulation frameworks. Destructive water has the limit of dissolving metals, fundamentally copper and lead, of the pipes framework, which accordingly builds the metal fixation in drinking water, prompting different wellbeing related issues.

Acidic water with pH under 7 is more destructive when contrasted with soluble water. Thus, treating the water with basic synthetic substances to build its pH is viewed as one of the most amazing proportions of decreasing water destructiveness.

Creation of Antacid Water

Antacid water can be created by water electrolysis that isolates acidic and soluble parts of water. Regular water that courses through rocks additionally accumulates minerals and becomes soluble in nature. Additionally, electrolyzed water can likewise be created from minerals, for example, calcium and magnesium, which are profoundly immersed with hydrogen.

This specific sort of water is known as basic decreased water.

Medical advantages of Antacid Water

Many investigations have asserted gainful wellbeing impacts of soluble water utilization. For example, it has been seen that oral organization of basic ionized water causes a decrease in blood levels of glucose, cholesterol, and fatty oil and works on metabolic working by smothering free extreme creation in mice that are prompted with metabolic turmoil. It additionally safeguards pancreatic beta cells from oxidative harms. In addition, antacid water assists in lessening the pace of weight with acquiring in corpulent mice by controlling cholesterol homeostasis.

In patients with end-stage renal illness, soluble water has been displayed to lessen unfriendly symptoms of hemodialysis, like over the top free extreme age. In the event of urinary bladder stone, basic water speeds up the discharge of melamine and forestalls its collection in the bladder, which thus further develops the neurotic circumstances related with bladder stone.

Since soluble water has higher pH, its innate limit of killing acids in the stomach settles on it a decent decision for treating gastrointestinal lot issues, like gastric hyperacidity, the runs, and so on. In instances of laryngopharyngeal and gastroesophageal reflux sicknesses, soluble water has displayed to irreversibly inactivate pepsin, an endopeptidase liable for reflux illness, by killing corrosive in the stomach.

In the event of activity prompted drying out in sound grown-ups, electrolyzed basic water has displayed to decrease the high-shear blood thickness, a coefficient to characterize gooey properties of blood.

Strangely, utilization of antacid water has additionally shown valuable impacts in advancing life span. Mice directed with antacid water have shown better endurance rate when contrasted with their partners that are controlled with customary water.

Other than potential medical advantages of drinking antacid water, washing with it likewise further develops skin-related issues. For instance, washing mice with soluble water has displayed to lessen skin harm related with UV radiation by keeping up with the harmony among supportive of and mitigating cytokines.

Is there any Gamble?

Notwithstanding many benefits of drinking soluble water, a legitimate quality control is fundamental to keep up with its pH inside physiologically OK reach. As per the WHO rules for drinking water quality, antacid water with pH more prominent than 9 causes skin and eye disturbance in mice and bunnies. In people, water with pH higher than 10 causes skin, eye, and bodily fluid film bothering; it might likewise actuate gastrointestinal disturbance in delicate people. Aside from these issues, cathode debasement during the course of water electrolysis may likewise produce exceptionally responsive platinum nanoparticles, which may likewise make poisonous impacts.

Figuring out acids and antacids

In unadulterated water, a little part of the atoms lose one hydrogen from the H2O structure, in a cycle called separation. The water hence contains few hydrogen particles, H+, and lingering hydroxyl particles, Goodness .

There is a harmony between the consistent development and separation of a little level of water particles.

Hydrogen particles (Goodness) in water get together with other water atoms to frame hydronium particles, H3O+ particles, which are all the more generally and just called hydrogen particles. Since these hydroxyl and hydronium particles are in harmony, the arrangement is neither acidic nor antacid.

A corrosive is a substance which gives hydrogen particles into arrangement, while a base or salt is one which takes up hydrogen particles.

All substances that contain hydrogen are not acidic as the hydrogen should be available in an express that is effectively delivered, dissimilar to in most natural mixtures which dilemma hydrogen to carbon molecules firmly. The pH in this way assists with measuring the strength of a corrosive by showing the number of hydrogen particles it discharges into arrangement.

Hydrochloric corrosive is areas of strength for an in light of the fact that the ionic connection between the hydrogen and the chloride particles is a polar one which is effectively broken down in water, producing numerous hydrogen particles and making the arrangement emphatically acidic. To this end it has an extremely low pH. This sort of separation inside water is likewise entirely positive as far as vivacious addition, which is the reason it works out with such ease.

Powerless acids are intensifies which in all actuality do give hydrogen however not promptly, like a few natural acids. Acidic corrosive, tracked down in vinegar, for example, contains a great deal of hydrogen however in a carboxylic corrosive gathering, which holds it in covalent or nonpolar bonds.

Accordingly, only one of the hydrogens can leave the particle, and all things being equal, there isn't a lot of security acquired by giving it away.

A base or salt acknowledges hydrogen particles, and when added to water, it absorbs the hydrogen particles framed by the separation of water so the equilibrium shifts for the hydroxyl particle focus, making the arrangement basic or fundamental.

An illustration of a typical base is sodium hydroxide, or lye, utilized in making cleanser. At the point when a corrosive and a soluble base are available in precisely equivalent molar focuses, the hydrogen and hydroxyl particles respond promptly with one another, creating a salt and water, in a response called balance.

What Is Antacid Water?

Water is vital to each cell, tissue, and organ in your body. The most ideal way to remain hydrated: glug-glug glasses of water over the course of the day.

Yet, which sort of water? Certain individuals guarantee that basic water is superior to whatever you might get from the tap. However, the science isn't there to back it up.

What Makes Soluble Water Unique?

Water is a mix of hydrogen and oxygen. That is the reason you call it H2O. Water's pH level decides how acidic it is and goes from 0 to 14. A pH of 7 is viewed as impartial. That "seven" number is viewed as impartial or adjusted among acidic and soluble. In the event that water is under 7 on the pH scale, it's "acidic." Assuming it's higher than 7, it's "soluble."

EPA rules express that the pH of faucet water ought to be somewhere in the range of 6.5 and 8.5. In any case, faucet water in the U.S. will in general fall underneath that - - in the 4.3 to 5.3 territory - - contingent upon where you reside.

Filtered water falls under various principles relying upon whether it professes to be basic. Packaged basic water has a pH level over 7. At times, producers utilize a unique gadget to change the synthetic cosmetics of the water. Different times, they add supplements to the water to change its pH.

For correlation, squeezed orange has a pH of 3.3 and dark espresso is around a 5. Unadulterated water has an unbiased pH of 7. Be that as it may, faucet water in the U.S. will in general fall underneath that - - in the 4.3 to 5.3 territory - - contingent upon where you reside.

Checking the Wellbeing Cases

Soluble water fans guarantee that its expanded hydrogen gives more noteworthy hydration than ordinary water, particularly after a hard exercise.

Devotees of the stuff likewise say that customary drinking water with a pH under 7 makes an excess of corrosive in your blood and cells. They fault plain water's low pH for a wide range of medical conditions, from osteoporosis to malignant growth.

Water that is more basic apparently decreases corrosive in the circulatory system and:

Further develops digestion

Increments energy

Eases back maturing

Further develops assimilation

Lessens bone misfortune

Patrons of high-pH water say it additionally has the ability to starve malignant growth cells

Might Basic Water at any point Do This?

The wellbeing claims about antacid water are more about deals than science. There isn't a lot of examination to help them.

Additionally, your body, all alone, can keep your pH levels at a balanced. Your kidneys are your underlying filtration framework. They must adjust the corrosive levels in your body. On the off chance that your blood gets too acidic, your body brings it somewhere near breathing out more carbon dioxide.

Your stomach is the incredible balancer. Your gastric juices - - a mix of stomach related proteins and hydrochloric corrosive - - kill all that you eat and drink. Essentially, your stomach will re-ferment antacid water before it can do anything the wellbeing claims guarantee.

How Can It Taste?

Basic water might taste severe or not quite the same as your faucet water. This can likewise change the flavor of anything you use it in, similar to espresso or tea.

Is It Safe?

Except if you have a kidney illness, basic water represents no serious wellbeing gambles. The high pH could make your skin dry and irritated or cause a steamed stomach, yet entirely that is pretty much all.

Since it's protected, however, doesn't mean it does anything for you. For every one of the advantages of a fine looking specimen, top off at the tap.

Customary pH levels in your body

PH is an estimation of how acidic or soluble something is.

The pH esteem goes from 0-14:

Acidic: 0.0-6.9

Nonpartisan: 7.0

Antacid (or fundamental): 7.1-14.0

A large number of the soluble eating regimen propose that individuals screen the pH of their pee to guarantee that it's basic (more than 7) and not acidic (under 7).

Notwithstanding, it's vital to take note of that pH fluctuates enormously inside your body. While certain parts are acidic, others are antacid — there's no set level.

Your stomach is stacked with hydrochloric corrosive, providing it with a pH of around 1.5-2.0Trusted Source, which is profoundly acidic. This acridity is important to separate food.

Then again, human blood is in every case somewhat basic, with a pH of 7.35-7.45.Trusted Source When your blood pH drops out of the ordinary reach, it very well may be deadly whenever left untreated.

Nonetheless, this just occurs during specific infection states, for example, ketoacidosis brought about by diabetes, starvation, or liquor admission.

Synopsis

The pH esteem estimates a substance's sharpness or alkalinity. For instance, stomach corrosive is profoundly acidic, while blood is somewhat soluble.

Food influences the pH of your pee however not your blood

The pH of your blood needs to stay steady for you to remain solid, and your body has a few powerful methods for directing it.

Food will not normally cause a significant change in the pH of your blood. Nonetheless, food could changeTrusted Source the pH at any point worth of your pee — however the impact is to some degree variable.

Discharging acids in your pee is one of the primary waysTrusted Source your body manages its blood pH.

For instance, in the event that you eat a huge steak, your pee will turn out to be more acidic a while later as your body disposes of the metabolic waste.

Thusly, pee pH is an unfortunate mark of by and large body pH and general wellbeing. It can likewise be influencedTrusted Source by factors other than your eating routine.

Synopsis

Your body firmly controls blood pH levels. In solid individuals, diet doesn't essentially influence blood pH, however it can change pee pH.

Corrosive shaping food varieties and osteoporosis

Osteoporosis is an ever-evolving bone illness described by a reduction in bone mineral substance. It's especially normal among postmenopausal ladies and can radically expand your opportunity of fracturesTrusted Source.

The soluble eating regimen hypothesis guarantees that to keep a steady blood pH, your body takes basic minerals from unresolved issues acids from corrosive framing food varieties. This is known as the "corrosive debris speculation of osteoporosis," and infers that corrosive framing food sources can cause bone mineral thickness misfortune.

Nonetheless, this hypothesis disregards the capability of your kidneys and your lungs. The blood can containTrusted Source various acids, which are by the same token "metabolic" (fixed) or "respiratory" (unstable).

Fixed acids are discharged in the pee, though unstable acids are discharged by the lungs. One unpredictable corrosive is carbonic corrosive, which is shaped by the lungs as a component of your breathing interaction. This builds the corrosiveness of your blood.

The kidneys, in the mean time, are reabsorbing bicarbonate, which comes from the carbonic corrosive in the blood. This whole cycle opposes change to the pH to permit you to remain in the essential pH range forever.

The corrosive debris speculation likewise neglects the job of collagen lossTrusted Source in osteoporosis. Amusingly, low degrees of orthosilicic corrosive and L-ascorbic acid in your eating regimen are firmly connected to such collagen misfortune.

Remember that new logical evidenceTrusted Source proposes no connection between dietary corrosive and bone wellbeing. As a matter of fact, a high protein, corrosive shaping eating routine might be connected to all the more likely bone wellbeing because of expanded calcium maintenance and initiation of IGF-1 chemical.

Outline

Research doesn't uphold the hypothesis that corrosive shaping weight control plans hurt your bones. Protein, an acidic supplement, even is by all accounts gainful.

Sharpness and malignant growth

Before, far reaching audits on the connection between diet-prompted acidosis — or expanded blood causticity brought about by diet — and malignant growth presumed that there is no immediate linkTrusted Source.

Fresher researchTrusted Source proposes that there may be a connection between the corrosive in food and disease.

In any case, this exploration doesn't reflect blood sharpness. It is likewise indistinct if dietary corrosive burden authoritatively causes malignant growth. Truth be told, tests have likewise effectively developed disease cells in a basic environmentTrusted Source.

And keeping in mind that cancers fill quicker in acidic conditions, the growths make this corrosiveness themselves. Not the acidic climate makes disease cells, however malignant growth cells that establish the acidic climate.

Synopsis

There's no connection between a corrosive shaping eating regimen and disease. Disease cells additionally fill in antacid conditions.

Genealogical weight control plans and sharpness

Looking at the corrosive soluble hypothesis from both a transformative and logical viewpoint uncovers errors.

One review assessed that 87% of pre-farming people ate soluble eating regimens which shaped the focal contention behind the advanced antacid eating routine.

Remember that our distant predecessors lived in immeasurably various environments with admittance to assorted food sources. As a matter of fact, corrosive shaping eating regimens were more commonTrusted Source as individuals moved further north of the equator, away from the jungles.

www.ingramcontent.com/pod-product-compliance
Lightning Source LLC
Chambersburg PA
CBHW071108260726

48661CB00006B/2527